52 ways
to create an AIDS-free
WORLD

52 ways
to create an AIDS-free
WORLD

Donald E. Messer

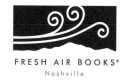

FRESH AIR BOOKS®
Nashville

52 Ways to Create an AIDS-Free World
Copyright © 2009 by Donald E. Messer
All rights reserved.

Fresh Air Books Web site: www.freshairbooks.org

FRESH AIR BOOKS® and design logos are trademarks owned by The Upper Room®, a ministry of GBOD®, Nashville, Tennessee. All rights reserved.

At the time of publication, all Web sites referenced in this book were valid. However, due to the fluid nature of the Internet, some addresses may have changed or the content may no longer be relevant.

Photographs are by Donald E. Messer, except photos used by permission of Sarah Harrington (pages 34, 42, 96); Pamela Merrill (page 26); John Blinn (pages 64, 80); Paul Jeffrey/Ecumenical Advocacy Alliance (page 52); Erik Alsgaard/United Methodist News Service (page 92); and International AIDS Society (page 110).

Cover design: iDesign, inc., Jay Arnold, graphic designer
First printing: 2009

LIBRARY OF CONGRESS CATALOGING-IN-PUBLICATION DATA
Messer, Donald E.
    52 ways to create an AIDS-free world / Donald E. Messer.
        p. cm.
    ISBN 978-1-935205-04-3
    I. AIDS (Disease)—Prevention. I. Title. II. Title: Fifty-two ways to create an AIDS-free world.
    RA643.8.M47 2009
    614.5'99392—dc22   2009001244

Printed in the United States of America

Fresh Air Books® is an imprint of Upper Room Books®

To my wonderful family

Bonnie J. Messer

Christine and Gordon Gallagher
and our grandchildren
Rachel, Noah, and Gabriel Gallagher

Kent Messer and Kate Hackett
and our grandchildren
Madeline and Eleanor Messer

Contents

III. A LACK OF CONSCIENCE

Introduction

NOBEL PEACE PRIZE WINNER Muhammad Yunus envisions in his book *Creating a World without Poverty* that someday humanity will build museums about poverty "to display its horrors to future generations." The Bangladeshi economist imagines that in the future people will "wonder why poverty continued so long in human society—how a few people could live in luxury while billions dwelt in misery, deprivation, and despair."[1]

Likewise, I dream of the day when museums will chronicle the emergence of a deadly virus called HIV and how the world successfully battled back to create an AIDS-free world. My recent visits to the apartheid museum in Johannesburg, South Africa, and the civil rights museum in Memphis, Tennessee, reminded me anew of the invaluable lessons to be learned from the struggles of those who suffered stigma and discrimination, as well as the sacrifices of those veterans of hope who effectively challenged the injustice of the status quo.

The time to construct such an institution to commemorate the end of AIDS is not yet; currently we are losing the battle to stop the pandemic. However, now is the time to discover ways to curtail and halt the global spread of this virus through education, prevention, research, care, and treatment.

Facing a Global Pandemic

Often described as the world's worst health crisis in seven hundred years, current statistical estimates indicate about 33.2 million people are HIV positive in the world; more than 25 million people have died from the disease. Some 2.5 million are children. Worldwide nearly 50 percent of those infected are women; in Africa 58 percent are women. About two-thirds of the globe's HIV-positive cases are in sub-Saharan Africa.

AIDS prevalence is increasing in Asia, with India having the second largest number of infections, just behind South Africa. China's numbers are escalating, and countries in Southeast Asia like Thailand, Cambodia, and Vietnam have significant numbers of persons infected. Likewise, Australia, Europe, Latin America, and the Caribbean face daily the challenges of this global pandemic.

In the United States more than one million persons are infected, but 25 percent do not know it because they have never been tested. Each year more than 52,000 new infections occur in the United States. Women represent 26 percent of all new cases. The disease especially affects women of color; AIDS is now the primary cause of death among African American women between the ages of 25 to 34. Seventy-two percent of all women were infected through heterosexual contact; 26 percent through drug use by injection.

In the face of this pandemic every person is called to take personal and social responsibility to help reverse the trends. The good news is that HIV and AIDS are preventable; the disease is not genetic and is not easily transmitted. The bad news is that neither a cure nor a vaccine exists, and none is likely soon. Therefore, prevention becomes a priority, and promoting care and treatment of persons infected and affected becomes a humanitarian imperative.

Why 52 Ways?

By using the imagery or strategy of fifty-two ways to correspond with the fifty-two weeks of the year, I intend to emphasize that the creation of an AIDS-free world requires not just the involvement of scientists, medical personnel, social workers, politicians, and other professionals but a daily commitment and engagement of persons from all walks of life.

Other books exist to help readers explore the HIV and AIDS pandemic in depth, but this short book of basic ideas makes an urgent appeal to people of all ages who wonder what they can do to make a difference.

I combine photos from my collection, quotations, and basic action statements with statistics and brief personal stories or illustrations that a reader can quickly assimilate. I draw upon my experiences in recent years as I have traveled extensively throughout the world, speaking and meeting with persons infected and affected by the disease. Since the journey from the mind to the heart is often the longest road, this book seeks not only to inform intellectually but also consciously to touch the human heart and move persons down the path to constructive action.

Since 2004 when my book *Breaking the Conspiracy of Silence* was launched in the House of Lords in London, England, I have been gratified to witness greater interest and involvement by government leaders and others in addressing this pandemic. Yet a dangerous apathy still exists on both a personal and social level that requires new vigilance in the battle to end HIV and AIDS in our lifetime. Since AIDS is a preventable disease, individuals can and do make a difference in reducing and eliminating the virus in the world.

This book calls persons of goodwill of many traditions, cultures, and countries to commitment and action. These persons can partner together to face a health hazard currently infecting more than 33 million people as well as millions more who are affected by the pandemic. Particular action points that I have advocated may prompt some persons to disagree, but that is to be expected because personal, religious, and political philosophies differ. My goal is not to be controversial or offensive but to be candid and provocative about how the world might become AIDS-free.

Unlike some books that claim there are only seven solutions for success or ten tasks to accomplish before becoming a millionaire, I recognize the arbitrariness of citing just fifty-two ways. I hope creative readers will expand this list, adding other practical suggestions.

By design this book does not require readers to read continuously from beginning to end; all topics related to stigma, prevention, treatment, and so on, are not placed together. Instead open the book at a topic that entices or a photo that appeals, and begin a journey of exploring what you can do to create an AIDS-free world.

Acknowledgments

Authors always are beneficiaries of the experiences, thoughts, and ideas of others. My travels around the world, speaking to individuals and groups engaged in addressing the global HIV and AIDS crisis, enrich my life. The stories that have been shared, and the struggles I have witnessed, are embedded in the fifty-two ways suggested in this book. To those countless individuals in Asia, Africa, and Latin America, often nameless but not faceless to me, I offer my profound thanks for their positive lives, despite often experiencing great adversity and poverty.

More specifically, I stand in debt to countless individuals who volunteer their vision, time, and energy to the work of the Center for the Church and Global AIDS, which I founded and serve as executive director. What an incredible experience to listen and to learn from these grassroots ambassadors of hope and health, love and life. When I began writing this volume, I solicited their ideas, many of which I have incorporated into the text. In particular, I want to express gratitude to Claudia Svarstad, Marla Petrini, Steve McCeney, Paula Murphy, M. Kent Millard, Jacob Kines, Jeff Corwin, Megan Armstrong, Shirley Snelling, Suzanne Calvin, Pam Merrill, Mary Loring, Kathryn Harris, Sarah Harrington, Julie White, Bill Graf, Kassie Seddon, Mandy Harkey, Kelly Triplett, Susan Brown, and Rhonda Dern; plus my son, Kent Messer, and daughter, Christine Gallagher.

An author's best friend is a critical editor. In my case, I have been blessed by more than one. Philip Miller of Denver provided invaluable insights and careful review of my initial manuscript. My wife, Bonnie, has encouraged the writing of these fifty-two ways from the very beginning, not only enduring the long hours apart while I wrote but also editing with the benefit of her considerable expertise as a psychologist and experience with AIDS around the world. To both Philip and Bonnie I express my heartfelt thanks.

Above all, I thank the editors of Upper Room Books for inviting this publication and for the creative imagination and professional editing skills of Kathleen Stephens, Robin Pippin, and Rita Collett.

Despite all this encouragement and assistance, ultimately I stand responsible for the final product. While I have made every effort to be accurate and comprehensive, I am certain to have missed some key dimensions in this complex pandemic. Therefore, I welcome written responses and ideas from readers at dmesser@iliff.edu or globalaids@gmail.com

I.

---

*If you judge people
you have no time to love them.*

— MOTHER TERESA

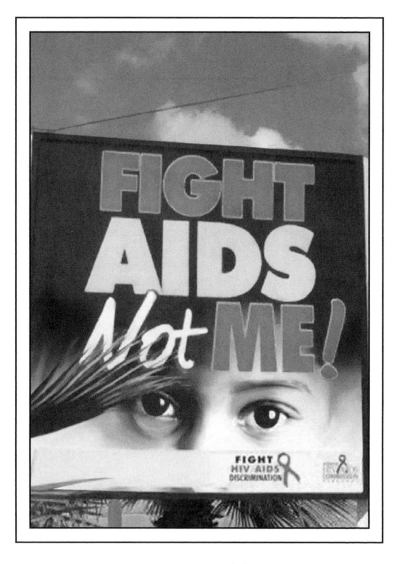

AIDS poster in Barbados

1 Hate the Disease, Not the People Infected

TOO OFTEN PEOPLE INFECTED with HIV are treated as pariahs, scorned by family, friends, and neighbors. Sometimes they have been thrown out of their homes or been violently attacked and killed. The virus is the enemy, not the people infected and affected. The disease does not spread easily or casually by sneezing, touching, or coughing, so it is safe to shake hands, hug, and share meals. If we imagine for a moment that we have just been diagnosed with HIV, what would we expect? Would we hope that family and friends would be supportive, or do we fear we would experience judgment, rejection, even shunning? How would people at work respond, or would we need to be secretive lest we lose a promotion or even our jobs? Is good health care available, or will we be left to the mercy of faceless government agencies and hostile health care workers? If we do not get treatment, how much will we suffer until the claws of death snatch us? What will happen to our children and loved ones? These are terrifying questions people around the world face as they learn they are among the six thousand newly infected daily. Asking "What if I had AIDS?" may remind us that the old-fashioned Golden Rule is not passé: "Do unto others as you would have them do unto you."

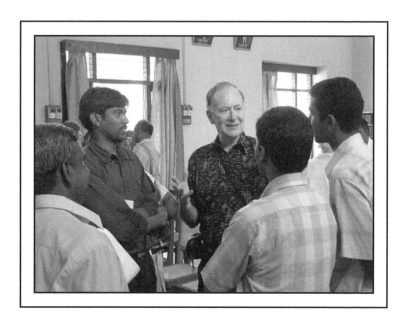

Students in India

2 Talk about AIDS

AIDS MAY NOT BE A dirty word, but it still tends to be more whispered than broadcast. If a family member is stricken by cancer or suffers a heart problem, people share freely and solicit sympathy. Cures for male erectile dysfunction now air regularly without embarrassment on radio and television during family sporting events and daily conservative talk shows. Prostate and breast cancer no longer hide in life's shadows. But because of the stigma associated with HIV and AIDS, silence prevails. While shopping recently, I encountered a store clerk who quietly confided that her brother was HIV positive. Unable to share this heartache with her store colleagues, sadly she could only trust me, a stranger, with her secret. By chatting about AIDS in caring and compassionate ways in our workplaces and among friends, we create an ethos that encourages openness, understanding, and acceptability.

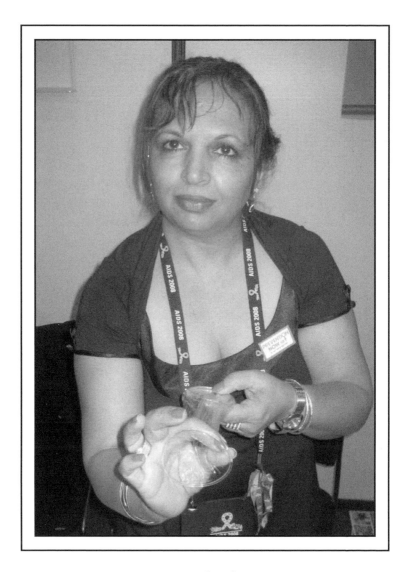

Demonstrating female condom in Mexico

3 Stop Having Sex

REFRAINING FROM SEXUAL relationships, or abstinence, obviously eliminates the possibility of getting HIV from sexual encounters. However, even the most ardent abstinence advocates rarely propose a radical universal prescriptive like stop having sex. They argue for maintaining abstinence from sex prior to and post-marriage. Abstinence encourages delayed sexual debuts, especially in countries where sexual encounters often begin as early as age twelve. What makes this virus so vicious is that HIV strikes at a basic human drive—the need for sex. If HIV were transmitted by something we eat—like apples or even chocolate—people could choose alternatives such as oranges or carob. Sex, fundamental both to baby making and loving human expression, has few alternatives. Stop having sex might be good counsel to discourage youthful sexual behavior but realistically once people begin having sex, few choose to quit. As a general maxim, stop having sex is neither practical nor utopian; a better way to state the caution is to shout: stop having *unprotected* sex!

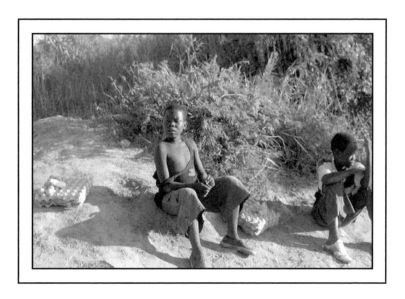

Boys selling eggs in Botswana

4 Make Hunger History

ABUNDANT FOOD EXISTS in the world, but every night over 900 million people go to bed hungry. The AIDS pandemic escalates the number of hungry people, since hunger ultimately causes AIDS and AIDS ultimately causes hunger. People without food often take desperate measures to feed themselves and their families. Women are often forced to sell their bodies. A twelve-year-old child in Haiti, involved in commercial sex work, was asked if she knew that she ran the risk of getting HIV and AIDS. The little girl answered, "I am afraid. But even if I get AIDS, I'll live a few years, won't I? You see, my family has no food for tomorrow." Working to make hunger history moves us closer to an AIDS-free world.

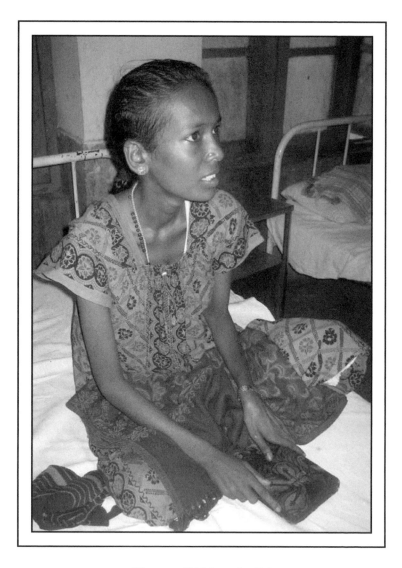

Woman in AIDS hospital in India

5   Emphasize Equality

THE WORLD RESERVES the worst stigmatization and discrimination for women. Gender inequality fuels the global AIDS pandemic. Nearly 50 percent of the persons infected worldwide are women; in sub-Saharan Africa the percentage hovers at 60 percent. Women are biologically, culturally, economically, politically, and religiously more susceptible to HIV. Because societies regard women as second- or third-class citizens, females often lack the power or right to control sexually even their own bodies, they rapidly succumb to the disease. The emergence of an AIDS-free world requires that both men and women emphasize equality and that laws ensure that no woman is treated inferior to a man. Most women are infected by their husbands or male partners. In many cultures, however, the women receive blame for spreading the disease and are often thrown out of their homes as they become victims of violence. The curbing of AIDS demands that we all become champions of equal rights—flaming feminists regardless of our gender!

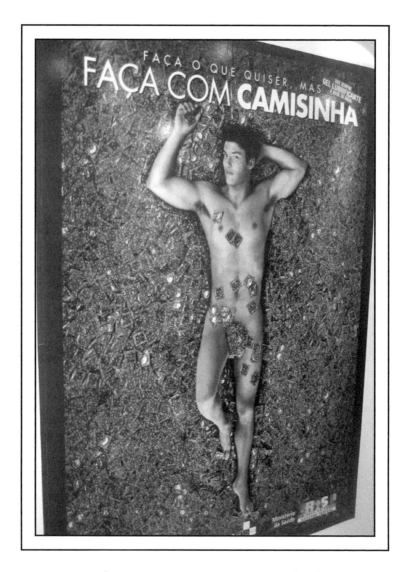

Brazilian prevention poster promoting safer sex with condoms

6 Be Frisky, Not Risky

HUMAN BEINGS ENJOY many ways of expressing their sexual feelings and energies. Ancient writings like the explicit *Kama Sutra* of India and antique sculptures from the early Greeks remind us that lovemaking in a variety of postures and places can be frisky and erotic. Modern-day bookstores are filled with volumes portraying in print and photos different positions couples may experiment with to enrich their sexual relationships. Magazine articles and talk show programs make clear that pleasure, not just procreation, is fundamental to the joy of sex. To be avoided, however, are risky behaviors like anal intercourse without a condom, sadomasochistic sex that involves blood or fluid exchange, or unprotected sex with a partner whose HIV status is unknown. A slogan might be "Enjoy but do not endanger—either yourself or your partner."

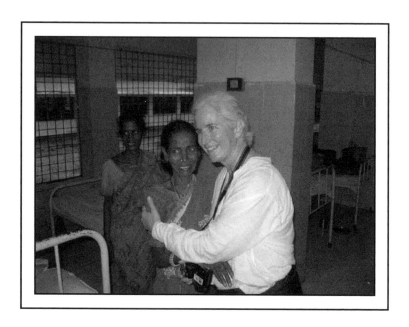

Embracing an AIDS patient in India

7 Befriend Persons Living with AIDS

ON AN AFRICAN TELEVISION channel, I saw an advertisement that contrasted ways people treat persons living with HIV and AIDS. A hospitalized man had his food shoved at him as if he were a dog; a contrasting scene showed college students embracing a young woman who had just learned she was HIV positive. The commercial's intent was not simply to promote humanitarian care but to lessen personal fears of disclosing HIV-positive status. If people feel confident that we are caring, accepting, and understanding persons, they will more likely share their burdens. The need for this TV campaign became quickly evident to me. The next day I met an abstinence-only educator who expressed surprise that a long-term colleague did not tell her she was HIV positive. I did not find it surprising since in just the hour I had been around this professor, I had heard her express self-righteous and judgmental statements. I would rather be sick and lonely than deal with her holier-than-thou presence. Healing care is not just the work of medical and social work professionals. By befriending persons infected and affected by HIV and AIDS in a nonjudgmental spirit, we bring hope and healing. As friends, we listen, touch appropriately, squeeze hands, give hugs, go to movies, invite persons to share a meal, and transport persons to the doctor's office. Such friendships inevitably prove mutually rewarding, as we discover anew the preciousness and precariousness of life.

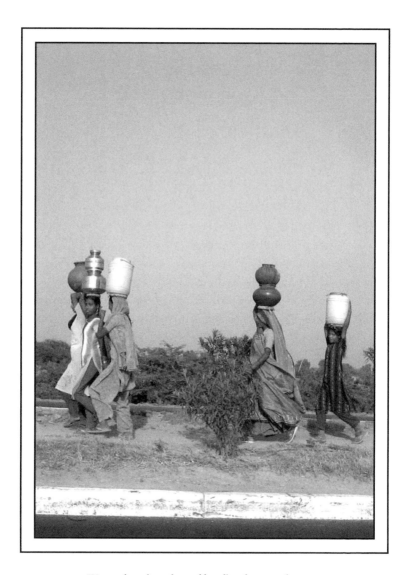

Women throughout the world walk miles to get clean water

8 Dig a Well

IF A GLASS OF CLEAN WATER was the only resource required to treat HIV and AIDS, the world could not deliver it to most people in need in sub-Saharan Africa. Globally women trek miles and miles every day in search of drinkable water to carry home on their heads for their families. Governments are beginning to distribute free antiretroviral medicines that do not cure HIV but make the disease more manageable. However, one billion people in the world lack safe drinking water, and 2.6 billion have inadequate sanitation. Taking powerful pills with contaminated water guarantees opportunistic infections that negate or complicate the effectiveness of the medicine. Persons already suffering from water-borne diarrheal diseases have weakened immune systems ripe for HIV infection. Former United Nations Secretary-General Kofi Annan said, "We shall not finally defeat AIDS, tuberculosis, malaria, or any of the other infectious diseases that plague the developing world until we have also won the battle for safe drinking water, sanitation, and basic health care." A visionary friend has set a goal of digging twenty wells in northern Malawi, mobilizing donors to help raise $10,000 for each project. A global campaign begins one aqua shaft at a time.

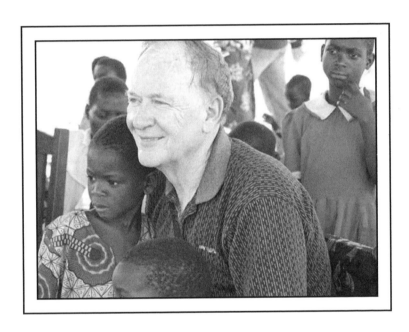

Caring for AIDS orphans in Malawi

9 Tackle the Taboos

EVERY CULTURE HAS ITS own set of traditional taboos prohibiting HIV prevention. "Polite" culture for centuries avoided tackling sexual taboos in particular because often they prompted personal embarrassment or conflicted with religious teachings. These cultures restrict communication about sex. At the close of one HIV workshop in India, the seminary president acknowledged that for the first time he might be able to talk candidly with his wife about sex. At a conference in Zambia an African woman challenged me during a lecture to put a condom on my thumb since she claimed those in the religious audience were too bashful to open the package. Expose whatever taboo is promoting death in your family or friendship circle, and dare to challenge the forbidden and prohibited.

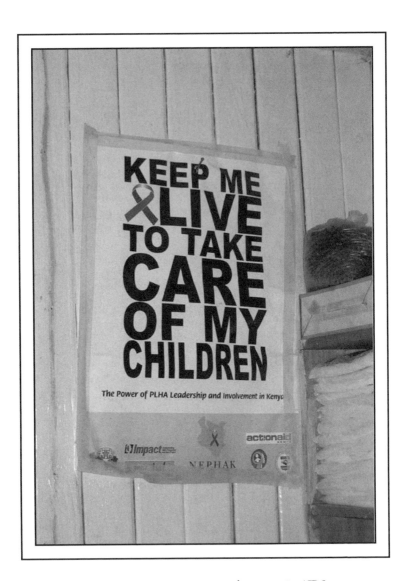

Kenya campaign urging testing and treatment for AIDS

10 Love Life

OPEN TO DIFFERENT interpretations, double entendres express two meanings, one often risqué. *Get Some* is the slogan for the New York City condom campaign. The double entendre, *loveLife* underscores two essential dimensions of an AIDS-free world. Its verbal imperative articulates a profound philosophy of cherishing life to its fullest. Or it can be an adjective describing one's personal sexual relationships and behavior. Either way, the slogan reminds us of the importance of self-respect and respect of the other if we are to create an AIDS-free world. Attentiveness to cultivating a culture that honors life and does nothing to inflict harm on anyone, particularly the weakest and most vulnerable, is critical to overcoming the AIDS pandemic. Self-protection against the virus is insufficient; love of partner and neighbor requires promoting safer sex practices and an ethos of gender equality, mutual consent, and protection against violence. In South Africa, where teenagers have a 50 percent chance of contracting HIV over the course of their lives, major AIDS campaigns now herald the slogan *loveLife* as a way to encourage prevention, care, and treatment.

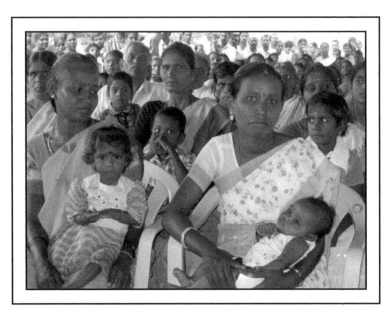

Mothers and children living with AIDS in India

11 Develop Microbicides

ALONG WITH A CURE or vaccines, scientists and public
health advocates dream of creating microbicides that
women can use to protect themselves against HIV.
Because women in many cultures and countries have little
or no control over their sexual lives, they yearn for freedom
to decide to prevent HIV. Men often stubbornly forbid the use
of condoms, even when they are HIV positive or have multiple
sexual partners. Women could apply this not-yet-developed
vaginal gel or cream prior to sexual intercourse without the
consent or knowledge of their male partner. Scientists predict that
microbicides would not be 100 percent effective, but more like 50
percent or 60 percent. But they would add one more weapon to
the arsenal in the fight against HIV and AIDS. Progress toward
this scientific breakthrough has been slow, with unexpected
setbacks and side effects. Microbicides, if manufactured for sale at
an inexpensive price, could be a revolutionary, nearly miraculous,
advance for the most impoverished women of the world.

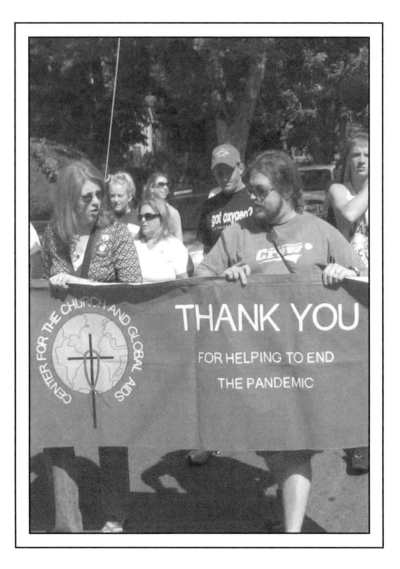

AIDS Walk in the United States of America

12 Walk, Even Sleep In, for Life

AROUND THE UNITED STATES, AIDS walks have become a primary method of raising funds to support civic and state organizations designed to battle the disease at the grassroots level. Donors pledge a given amount per mile hiked. Besides providing good exercise for participants and their families, these annual AIDS walks demonstrate a sense of solidarity in communities among those infected and affected. Every step forward we take, the better the probability that the message of AIDS prevention will be communicated. Government funding is never enough; private sources are needed to provide the necessary outreach programs of prevention, testing, counseling, nutrition, and care. In recent years, apathy has begun to prevail, and the traditional AIDS walks have yielded less income for agencies than in the past. Some have sought to stimulate charitable giving with Sleep-In campaigns, to encourage even the exhausted or the lazy to contribute to the cause. Everyone can participate, whether walking or sleeping, to promote prevention and preserve life, making sure invaluable community organizations get needed funding.

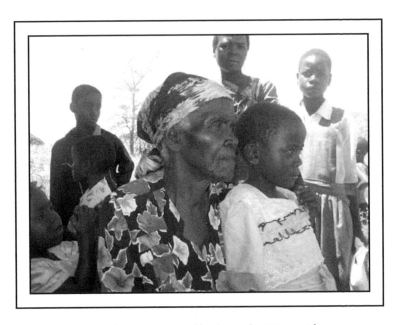

Grandmother caring for granddaughter with AIDS in Malawi

13 Partner with Grandparents

ONE DAY AN HIV-POSITIVE woman in rural Meru, Kenya, told me that her granddaughter could get free tuition for a secondary education, but "I can't even buy her a toothbrush, much less books and school clothing." That night the leader of an anti-AIDS network in this region handed me a list of more than 1,300 AIDS orphans, listing each by name, age, and gender. Globally more than 15 million children need care because one or both parents have died from the disease. Building orphanages to house all these little ones is both impossible and undesirable. Orphanages at their best are expensive to operate, move kids from their communities, and result in children who often suffer from emotional detachment. A better approach keeps families together by partnering with grandparents and other relatives and providing subsidies to help with costs of education, nutrition, and health. A yearly donation of $150 through the Gift of HOPE (Helping Orphans by Providing Essentials) via the Center for the Church and Global AIDS (www.churchandglobalaids.org) ensures a child's care and enables a continuing relationship with family and friends.

II.

In the fight against AIDS,
condoms save lives.
If you oppose the distribution of condoms,
something is more important to you
than saving lives.

—MELINDA GATES

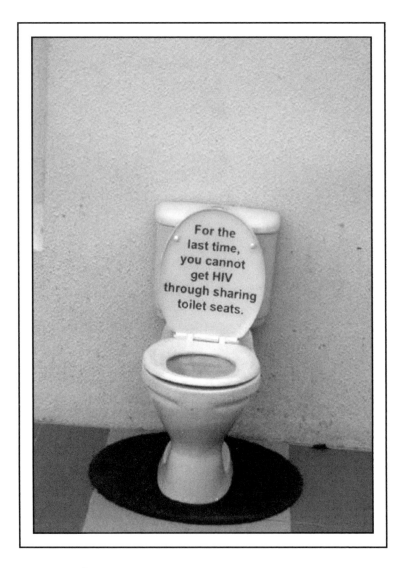

Advertising campaign against AIDS stigmatization in Singapore

14 Overcome "AfrAIDS"

FEAR CAN BE A HEALTHY stimulus to careful living. Fear prompts us to shun contaminated water, avoid dangerous neighborhoods, wear a seat belt, refuse tobacco products, sleep under a mosquito net, and pay our taxes. Fear of sexually transmitted diseases, including HIV, helps moderate our behavior and encourages safer-sex practices like using a condom and being faithful to one's partner. However, excessive and unwarranted fear can be detrimental to life. AfrAIDS, or the fear of AIDS, has led people to shun HIV-positive persons for fear of getting infected, even though the disease is not spread by coughing, handshaking, sharing food, hugging, or even light kissing. Overcoming the fear of AIDS allows both HIV-positive and negative persons to live, work, love, and partner together in the struggle to create an AIDS-free world.

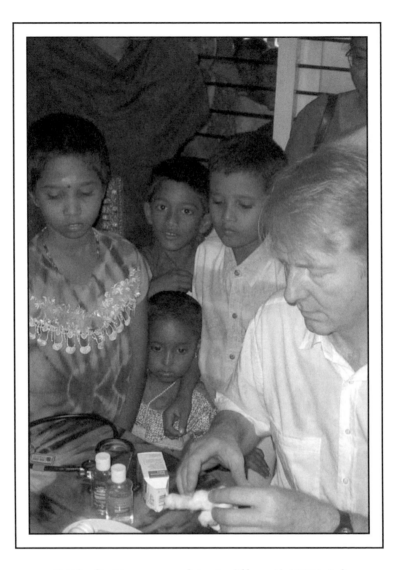

British pediatrician prepares medicines for children with AIDS in India

15 Stop Mother-to-Child HIV Transmission

HIV INFECTS MORE than 600,000 babies each year; 2.5 million children in the world live with HIV and AIDS. This insidious virus slips from mother to fetus in the womb or passes into the baby at birth or crosses to the child later through breast milk. Mother-to-child transmission causes 22 percent of the new HIV cases in Uganda. Some 420,000 children in India are infected each year. Failure to test pregnant women for the virus leads to the unintentional consequence of children being born with this life-threatening disease. If HIV-positive mothers are identified, they can receive an inexpensive pill at the time of childbirth, followed by a sip of antiretroviral syrup for the newborn baby. This medicine dramatically reduces the probability of an infected baby. When Lilian Akoth Juma, twenty-seven, learned she had HIV, she wanted to be sterilized but had no access to the procedures or to birth control. When her husband died, she was "inherited" by another man as dictated by local customs. Recently, when she gave birth to twins on her dirt-floor home in western Kenya, she received no pills and her babies no syrup. By finding ways to purchase and distribute medicine costing only 50 cents to one dollar, countless children can experience an AIDS-free life. The Elizabeth Glaser Pediatric AIDS Foundation (www.pedaids.org) helps provide this medicine. Church organizations like the United Methodist Global AIDS Fund also help. Donating can mean the difference between life and death.

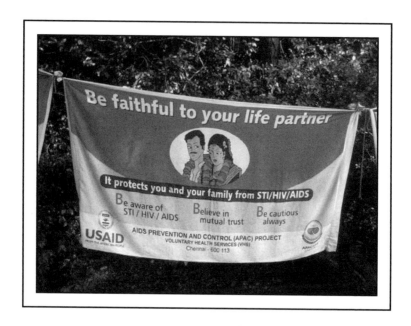

USAID poster in India

16 Practice Zero Grazing

OFTEN OVERLOOKED OR underemphasized in the famous ABC approach to AIDS prevention (A=abstinence, B=being faithful, C=consistent condom use) is the B dimension—being faithful to one's partner. In parts of Africa, multipartner relationships are common, helping to spiral the spread of HIV. Visits to sex workers by married men in India and elsewhere in Asia is common. Premarital, postmarital, and extramarital sex exist in many cultures and countries. The more sexual partners, the greater the probability of infection. Uganda significantly reduced its rate of infection after colorful billboard campaigns urged zero grazing, meaning: stick to one sexual partner. The efficacy of this prevention method depends upon the willingness of both partners in a sexual relationship to practice zero grazing. If one sexual cohort or both are checking to see if "the grass is greener" on the other side of the fence, then the risk of infection increases significantly. Mutual faithfulness is essential to guard against HIV.

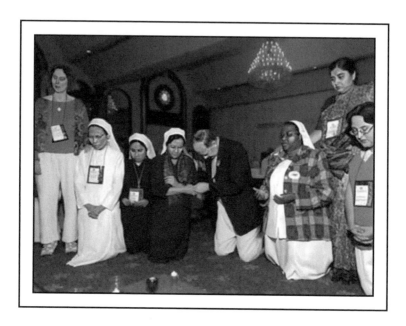

Praying at International AIDS Conference in Thailand

17 Pray

PEOPLE OF ALL religious faiths around the world pray and meditate. In Bangkok, Thailand, at the fifteenth International AIDS Conference, for the first time in this conference's history, religious leaders from all the major religions—Muslim, Christian, Hindu, Buddhist, and Jewish—gathered to lift their voices together to the Holy. Prayer brings comfort to the sick and encouragement to the suffering. Tearful prisoners with AIDS in a locked hospital ward in India unexpectedly crawled off their beds and knelt before me, pleading for prayer, even though we did not share the same language. Shaken, I did the best I could, trusting divine powers beyond me. Pray daily for those infected and affected by HIV and AIDS. Express hopes for a future cure and vaccine. Prayer is neither a panacea for good judgment nor a prophylactic for risky behavior, but meditation can provide clarity and courage when we face difficult personal dilemmas and choices.

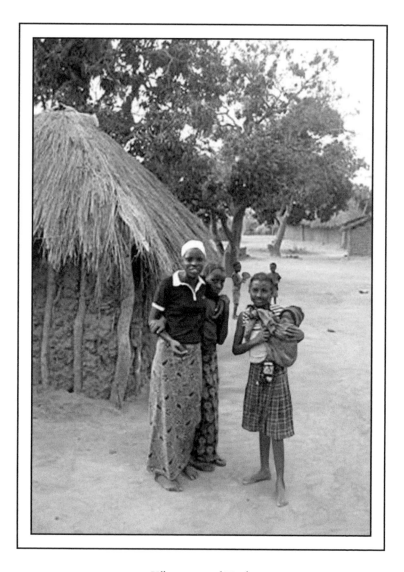

Villagers in rural Zambia

18 Question Unhealthy Cultural Traditions

CULTURAL RELATIVISM is popular in some intellectual circles. Some deeply rooted, societal traditions encourage tolerance and respect. An AIDS-free world, however, requires challenging certain cultural traditions like widow cleansing, practiced in parts of sub-Saharan Africa. When a man dies, the mourning wife is expected, if not compelled, to have sexual intercourse with his older brother or a professional community cleanser. Since either person might be HIV positive, this atypical practice is ripe for spreading the virus. Myths, like the idea of having sex with a young virgin cures HIV, have led to widespread child abuse. Likewise, other traditions, such as the marriage of young girls, the use of unsterile knives in circumcision, demand for dry vaginal sex, and inadequate sex education cry out for reexamination. Stemming the pandemic means not only questioning these cultural patterns but insisting they be stopped.

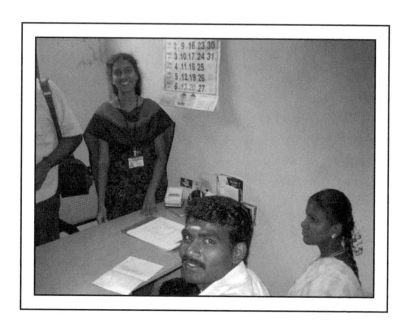

Counseling at a rural health clinic in India

19 Encourage Volunteer Counseling and Testing

A FRIEND IN MALAWI reports that he and his fiancée visited the volunteer counseling and testing center prior to getting their marriage license. Knowing each other's HIV status enables persons to make informed decisions about their relationship. Testing is not an absolute guarantee, since the virus can remain latent for three to six months before showing up in a test. However, the testing and counseling process itself can be a helpful educational step for couples. If one or both persons test positive, then counseling can help a couple make personal and family planning decisions. Persons who test negative for the virus need not think they are forever immune. Practicing safer-sex methods and avoiding contaminated needles remain imperative. Rather than despair, a person who tests positive for HIV can seek counseling and medical help. Modern medicines do not cure but do offer hope and opportunities for managing the disease and for positive living.

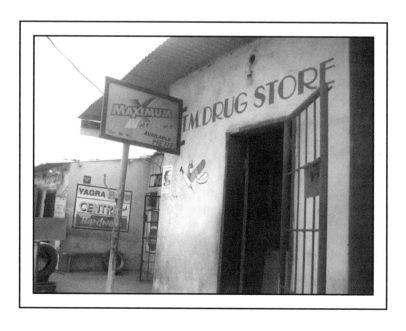

Pharmacy in Zambia advertising Maximum condoms

20 Call for PEP in an Emergency

PEOPLE MAKE MISTAKES; accidents happen; sexual violence occurs. Sometimes sexual passion overrules judgment, or alcohol and drugs blind decision making, prompting unprotected sex with an HIV-positive partner. A medical professional's needle slips, and he or she gets infected with contaminated blood. A woman or man is raped. In these circumstances there is hope of preventing infection, thanks to postexposure prophylaxis (PEP) treatment. If two antiretroviral drugs are administered within seventy-two hours of an exposure, the risk of contracting the virus diminishes considerably. However, the unpleasant negative side effects like prolonged fatigue and extreme nausea make this toxic treatment unpopular. PEP is not universally accessible, even in the United States, because some public officials fear it encourages risky behavior— the same argument used against condom distribution or abortions. Yet one study of PEP recipients actually showed that over the following year they had a 73 percent decrease in high-risk sexual behavior. Like treatment for gunshot wounds or stabbings, PEP should be available in an emergency to all who need it. If you or a friend faces an emergency, don't just call 911, call for PEP!

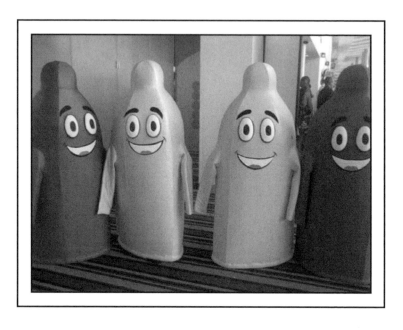

Cartoon condoms at Mexico International AIDS Conference

21 Thank God for Condoms

CONDOMS, USED CORRECTLY and consistently, are
humanity's best protection against getting infected by
HIV while engaging in vaginal, oral, or anal sex. All sexual
behavior involves a degree of risk, so practicing safer sex
using condoms is imperative. Condoms are deemed to be the
greatest "weapon of mass protection" available; without them
millions more people would be infected each year. Is that not a
good reason to thank the Divine?

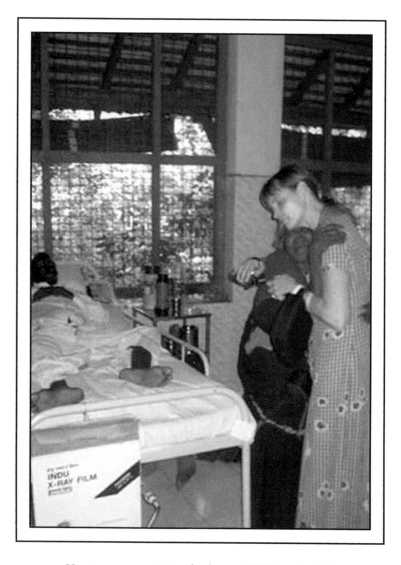

Hugging woman caring for a loved one in AIDS hospital in India

22 Oppose Double Standards

IF WE WANT TO WIPE HIV and AIDS off the earth, then we must eliminate current double standards governing gender behavior. In many African countries, current double standards encourage boys to get an education, while girls stay at home to help with household duties. Girls, often forced into early marriages, may experience dreadful domestic violence. Married men, particularly in Asia, commonly visit commercial sex workers, helping to spur the pandemic. Macho men refuse to use condoms, despite the wishes of their female partners. If a woman has the option of a female condom, the man often rejects the request, accusing her of promiscuity, even while knowing that he is the one who has engaged in risky extramarital behavior. Double standards prevail in terms of HIV and AIDS care and treatment as well. In an Indian AIDS hospital, I have seen mothers, daughters, and wives caring for sick husbands, fathers, and brothers. In the same hospital I have visited sick women and discovered they are dying alone.

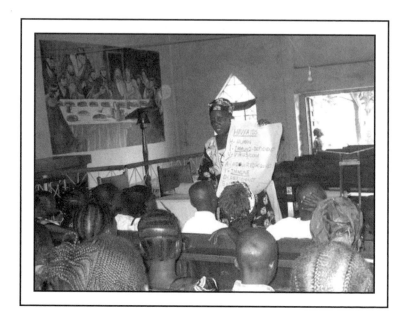

Teaching children about AIDS in Sierra Leone

23 Teach Children about Sex and AIDS

SEX EDUCATION GETS a bad rap. The fear of undercutting parenting rights and introducing inappropriate ideas to children prompts some to silence responsible efforts to communicate basic information about sexual health. Even those who favor educating young people about sex and AIDS find themselves embarrassingly inarticulate at times, not knowing what is age-appropriate information. However, if parents, teachers, and counselors fail to teach children about sexual health, kids will learn from peers or search the Internet for answers to their questions. Many African communities have learned that their efforts to teach children came too late; sexually active youth were already HIV positive. Strangers should not be telling children there is no Santa Claus or introducing an uninvited "birds-and-bees" lecture. Each of us, however, has to find ways to communicate about sex and AIDS within the context of our family values. Let us take responsibility to ensure that the community has ways to educate young people whose parents and guardians fail to equip them for a safe and healthy life.

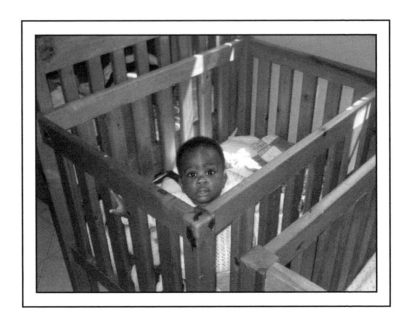

Baby with AIDS in Zambia awaiting adoption

24 Fight for Peace

FIGHTING FOR PEACE SOUNDS like an oxymoron equivalent to *jumbo shrimp*, *military intelligence*, and *airline service*. Yet the combative language may signify a greater urgency for reducing civil conflicts and minimizing wars than more pacifist verbiage. HIV and AIDS have become weapons of war in civil conflicts in the Congo, Sudan, Sierra Leone, and Liberia, as soldiers plunder and rape. Refugee camps, overrun with desperate women and children, are especially vulnerable to the pandemic. Even United Nations peacekeepers have been found guilty of spreading the virus from country to country. Wars destroy the social structures that bond people and communities together, disrupt educational programs, and undermine the moral fabric of societies. AIDS cannot be conquered in a world at war.

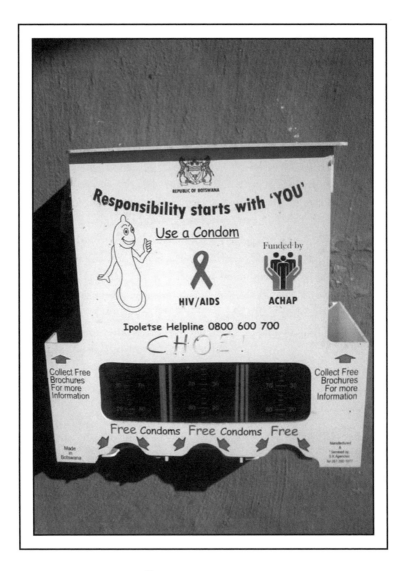

Botswana prevention program

25 Buckle Up

In Africa, Asia, and Latin America, it's nearly impossible to get people to buckle up car safety belts. In America, personal liberty champions often resent and resist using helmets while riding motorcycles. Whole families dangle precariously on motor scooters in India. We witness risky personal behavior daily on the roads of the world. When risk-taking behavior of all types is the norm for so many, it is little wonder that advocating caution such as sexual abstinence or the correct and consistent use of condoms meets such resistance. In a striking advertisement aimed at young men, a variety of tablets used for treating HIV and other opportunistic diseases are displayed. The tagline declares, "If you think a condom is bothersome, try taking twelve pills a day!" Benjamin Franklin's old proverb is worth remembering: "An ounce of prevention is worth a pound of cure." Especially when there is no cure.

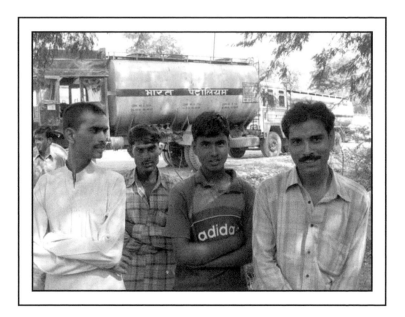

Truck drivers in India

26 Get Checked Regularly for STDs

SEXUALLY ACTIVE PERSONS outside a monogamous relationship are at greater risk of contracting sexually transmitted diseases (STDs). Common STDs like syphilis, gonorrhea, chlamydia, and genital warts can be cured if detected and treated early. Others like herpes and HIV can be controlled but not cured. STDs weaken the immune system, which allows HIV to move in more readily. Thus, regular checkups and quick treatment eliminate the spread of STDs, including HIV. Abstaining from sex or practicing protected sex are the best ways to avoid or reduce the possibility of infecting others. Stopping the spread of STDs must be both a personal priority and a public health imperative.

III.

The HIV/AIDS crisis is
not a crisis of lack of resources.
It is a crisis of lack of conscience.
It is the obscene gap between
the haves and the have nots
that is driving this holocaust.

—People Living with HIV/AIDS
in Lusaka, Zambia

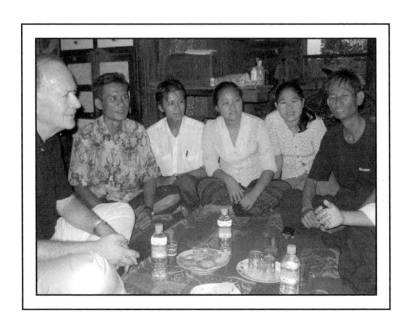

Sharing food with persons living with AIDS in Myanmar (Burma)

27 Speak Out against Stigma

FAMILY MEMBERS PRESSURED Grandma not to invite her grandson to the annual Thanksgiving reunion because he recently had been diagnosed HIV positive. They threatened not to attend, expecting that she would reconsider in light of the prospect of the family's boycotting her favorite event. Grandma, however, spoke out clearly, "The doors of my home are open to all of my family. My grandson will always be welcomed at my table." Because she spoke out against stigmatization in favor of inclusion, the grandson not only was present, but every other member of the family also attended and learned a lesson in acceptance.

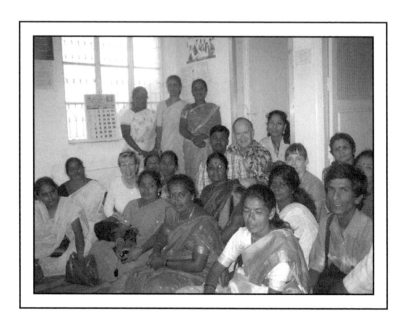

Meeting to discuss challenges faced by commercial sex workers in India

28   Decriminalize Sex

PUBLIC HEALTH OFFICIALS around the world are
handcuffed by harassing laws that penalize same-sex
relationships. Colonialism left antisodomy laws sprinkled
throughout the world—in places like Kenya, India,
Bangladesh, Jamaica, Barbados, Singapore, and Zambia.
Religious restrictions encourage the criminalization of
homosexuality in Egypt, Indonesia, Nigeria, and many other
countries. Endless controversies rage almost everywhere over the
legalization of commercial sex work. Children and youth must be
protected by law from pedophiles and sexual violence. Agencies
struggle to launch AIDS-prevention advertising campaigns
targeted to sex workers or to men who have sex with men in
countries where such relationships are illegal. Significant segments
of the population are overlooked when fear keeps persons from
seeking testing and counseling. Few people believed the president
of Iran when he declared, "We don't have homosexuals, like in
your country." What is believable is that people are forced to lead
double sexual lives, lest the government choose to enforce
draconian laws regulating private behavior. Criminalization
policies tend to negate HIV educational efforts aimed toward
at-risk groups and provide stumbling blocks to creating an
AIDS-free world.

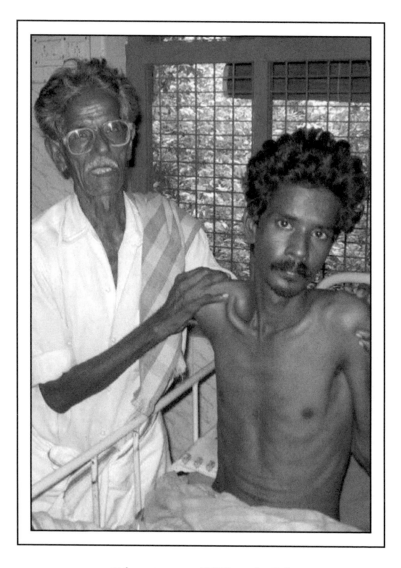

Father assists son in AIDS hospital in India

29 Beware of Blood Contaminators

IF VAMPIRES WERE the primary way persons were infected with HIV, the world would have no reason to worry. But HIV is not spread by mosquito bites or bloodsucking bats, and only rarely when an infected person accidentally bites another. We need not fear these vermin or accidents as they relate to HIV infection. What *does* significantly spread the disease are contaminated blood supplies, like bad blood transfusions that plagued the U.S. system in the mid-1980s but were left uncontrolled and unacknowledged in China's Henan Province for many years. Drug addicts who reuse syringes are a major source of new infections in places like Eastern Europe, Southeast Asia, and the United States. Mitigation of the potential dangers and health risks of contaminated blood requires new strategies. Harm-reduction efforts include needle exchange programs or supervised injection sites for intravenous drug users. Critics fear these efforts facilitate dangerous behavior. However, studies demonstrate that drug use does not increase with needle exchange and supervised injection sites—but the spread of HIV and hepatitis is reduced.

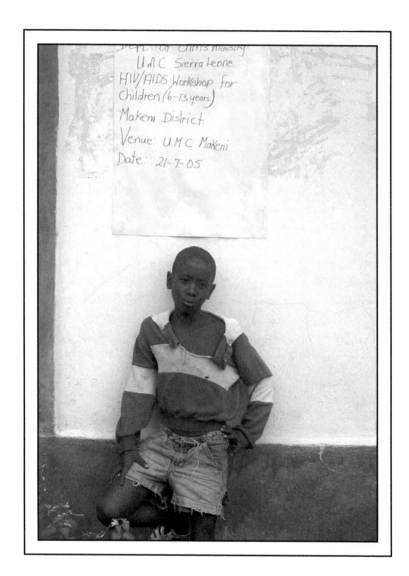

Young boy in Sierra Leone

30 Change the World with Pocket Change

Six-year-old Marie and her parents watched a television special that focused on AIDS in Africa. When the program finished, her parents switched off the set, and returned to that day's activities. But Marie interrupted with a question, "What are we going to do?" Startled, they responded, "What do you mean, what are we going to do?" Persistent, Marie persuaded her parents to drop their daily pocket change into a large jar. Later she took her cause to her small local church. As a result, $2,000 worth of pocket change helped a dozen AIDS-impacted children in Sierra Leone get care and attend school that year.

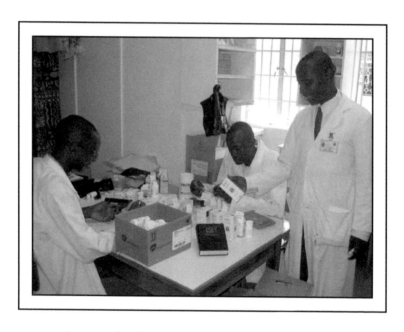

Antiretroviral medicine from the United States being sorted in Kenya

31 Treat More People— Prevent More Infection

MORE AGGRESSIVE EFFORTS to treat persons with HIV could reduce future AIDS cases by as much as 60 percent. Powerful antiretroviral drugs not only lengthen the life of patients but also dramatically reduce the severity of the virus, making it less likely that they will infect others. Advocates argue that expanded treatment will save tens of millions of dollars in future public health-care costs since fewer people will be infected. Skeptics fear that infected persons who think they are "cured" may engage in risky sexual behavior, forgetting good prevention methods. Costs of medication and potential side effects also make people hesitant about starting treatment. However, Julio Montaner, M.D., President of the International AIDS Society, argues that "bottom line . . . no matter how you configure it, the more people you treat, the more infections you prevent."[2]

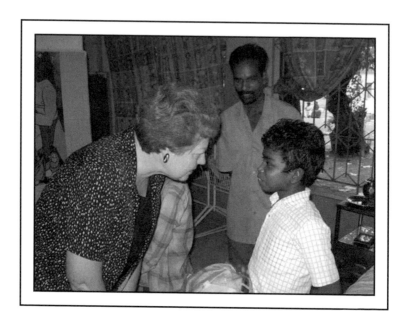

Greeting a child in an AIDS hospital in India

32 Respect and Promote Confidentiality

WHEN RUMORS SPREAD and confidentiality was broken, a young Burmese couple discovered persons boycotted their little tea and soup shop in Yangon. When a seminary student in northeast India was exposed as being HIV positive, the faculty threw him out of school immediately; in despair, he committed suicide. In South Africa young men avoid testing because they do not trust professionals to keep confidences and respect their privacy. Broken confidences subject persons to stigmatization, discrimination, and sometimes even violence. Gossip creates a hostile climate by discouraging testing and counseling. This cycle of broken confidentiality, fear, and stigma helps fuel the global HIV pandemic. Lest lack of confidentiality be a cloak for irresponsibility, persons testing HIV positive have an ethical and, in some cases, legal responsibility to protect others by informing sex partners of their status, avoiding unprotected sex, and not donating contaminated blood. Critical to attacking AIDS is respecting and promoting the human right to confidentiality.

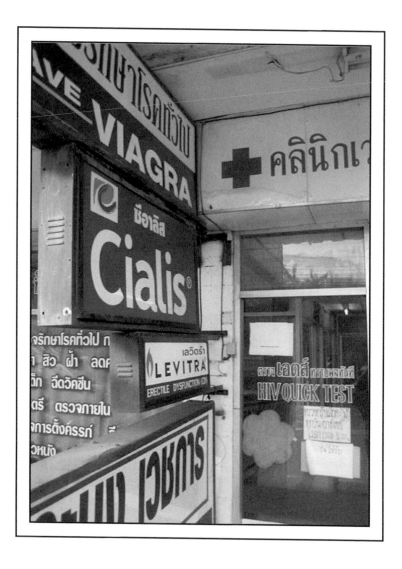

Advertising both AIDS testing and erectile dysfunction pills in Thailand

33 Masturbate

MASTURBATION—A WORD that makes liberals blush, conservatives angry, and libertarians flinch! Widely practiced but rarely discussed in polite company, this way of avoiding HIV needs to be underscored. Self-stimulation sexually eliminates any chance of infection, and mutual masturbation between partners is a very low risk sexual activity, unless one person has open sores or cuts. Yet when the United States Surgeon General Joycelyn Elders proposed teaching youth about masturbation as part of AIDS education, she lost her job. We do not like to hear about such things. The world would have less HIV and AIDS today if more men chose to masturbate instead of visiting commercial sex workers. In most cultures and countries, embarrassment triumphs over public health policy, so this topic remains taboo.

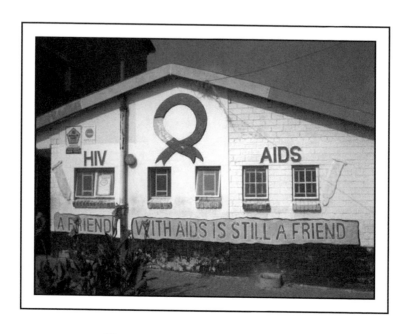

Middle school in South Africa teaching AIDS prevention

34 Think Twice about Mixing Alcohol and Sex

THE USE AND ABUSE of alcohol remains an underreported dimension of the global AIDS pandemic. Headlines blare reports of teenage drinking, resulting in out-of-control parties and tragic car accidents. But because AIDS has a long incubation period, what resides below the surface is how adolescent drinking mixed with sex often results in an AIDS diagnosis years later. Evidence suggests that heavy drinking among people of all ages has a direct correlation to increased rates of HIV infection. Chronic alcohol consumption does not increase susceptibility to HIV or accelerate AIDS, but alcohol can impact an individual's inhibitions and decision making. Under the influence, persons might choose sexual activities that they would otherwise forego. Heavy and frequent drinkers tend to engage in more impulsive sexual behavior, more often use injecting drugs, and have more unprotected sex. Heavy drinkers use condoms less frequently, thereby increasing their chances of infection. So think twice about mixing alcohol and sex, since this combination often leads to unsafe sex. Interventions that reduce alcohol abuse and dependency can significantly improve the success of global HIV preventive and treatment strategies.

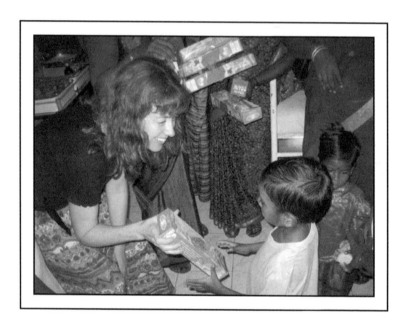

Sharing a gift with an AIDS orphan in India

35 Volunteer Time and Donate Money

AIDS ORGANIZATIONS AROUND the world have slim
staff, unstable income sources, and a backlog of requests
for service. Glamor is rarely attached to grassroots AIDS
volunteer work. Involvement in the struggle against AIDS
on a local level does not land the volunteer on the society
page of the local newspaper. People handing out condoms on a
street corner or addressing newsletters in a crowded room or
delivering food to homebound AIDS patients seldom receive the
mayor's award for humanitarian service. Telling your friends or
neighbors that you volunteer for a local AIDS organization may
invite more suspicion than praise. Not everyone can head for
Rwanda to work in an AIDS orphanage or to Honduras to offer
medical care to women in a shantytown. Spending time, energy,
and resources through volunteer efforts either locally or
internationally not only benefits persons living with HIV and
AIDS but also tends to deepen and transform the volunteer's
perspectives and commitment regarding the global pandemic.

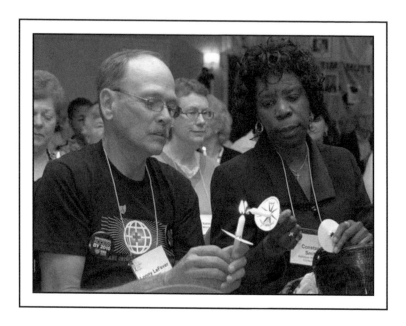

Memorial AIDS service in the United States of America

36 Observe World AIDS Day

EACH YEAR ON DECEMBER first, persons around the globe observe World AIDS Day. A day set aside to remember the more than 25 million people who have died since the pandemic began, it is also a time for renewed educational efforts promoting prevention, care, and treatment. Each year UNAIDS releases the latest global statistics about the extent and trends of the pandemic. These statistics are only estimates; an exact count is impossible for many reasons: government unwillingness in some countries to share information; lack of medical infrastructure to gather accurate data; and the tendency for people to deny the real reason a person has died, since dying from AIDS may be treated as a stigma for survivors. Attend or plan a World AIDS Day observance. Do not be surprised if attendance is low, since many people prefer not to be reminded of the reality of what public health experts call the worst health crisis in seven hundred years. Find a strategy to break through this wall of apathy. Consider writing a letter to the editor of your local newspaper, creating a public informational display, or getting involved in a demonstration that attracts the media and awakens the citizenry.

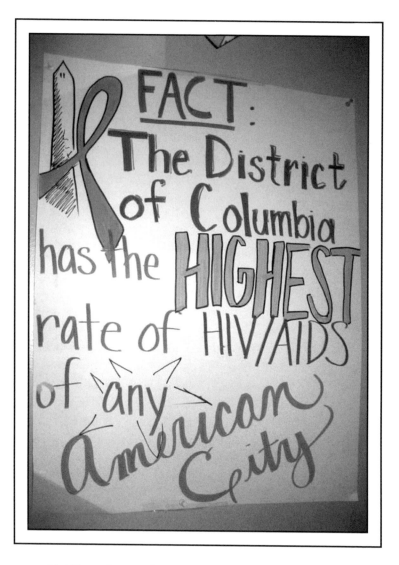

The US capital city, Washington, DC, has 3 percent HIV prevalence rate

37 Avoid Dangerous, Illegal Drugs

THE TEMPTATION TO experiment with dangerous, illegal drugs is not confined to one culture or country. Often people do not realize how use of these substances increases their probability for becoming infected with HIV. In rural Kenya I discovered a high rate of AIDS in a region where people regularly chewed on twigs of trees that grow abundantly in the region. Ingesting miraa, a mild stimulant herb, dulls decision-making abilities, leading to unwise and unsafe sexual behavior. In the United States addiction to smoking tobacco or snorting methamphetamine (also called speed, ice, or glass) affects the brain, causing confused thinking and lowered sexual inhibitions. Worldwide a small pill or powder called ecstasy causes a warm, loving feeling, making people more willing to have sex. The peril of overdosing and the damage to the human body make these drugs not only dangerous but also deadly. Avoidance and abstinence from these products is essential to curb and conquer AIDS.

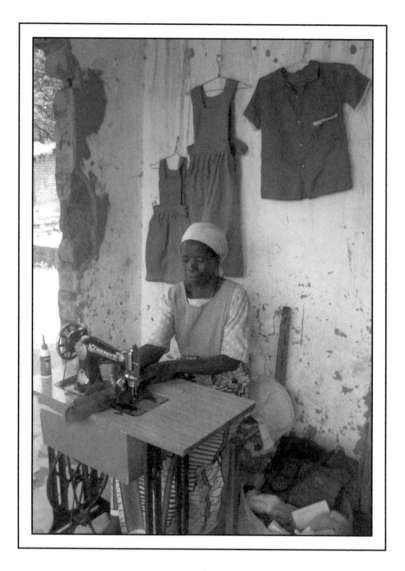

Income-generating business in Malawi

38 Start a Social Business

IMPOVERISHED PEOPLE WITH HIV and AIDS will never escape the misery-go-round of ill health, poor education, and poverty with only the help of charities or even government. Nobel Peace Prize winner Muhammad Yunus of Bangladesh contends that one way to eradicate poverty is through social businesses that enable persons to become self-supporting. Philanthropic entrepreneurs can start up social businesses that recover their investment, then provide profits to pursue charitable goals. For example, women concerned with educating AIDS orphans are exploring the introduction of Western-style quilt-making to Kenya. Quilts with an African theme have great potential market value in Europe and the United States. Another vision involves weaving colorful Indian saris into attractive wall hangings that would sell in the U.S. market and benefit a rehabilitation program for commercial sex workers in South India (onemother.org). Creating microcredit programs for the poor who lack collateral provides yet another option. This strategy allows persons to start their own profit-making business, eventually earning enough to pay back the loans. With a microcredit loan, one African woman with AIDS began raising corn on her little plot of land to feed her family and soon expanded into a profitable and sustainable business that employed others who were HIV positive. Self-sustaining people do not rely on donors who may experience compassion fatigue.

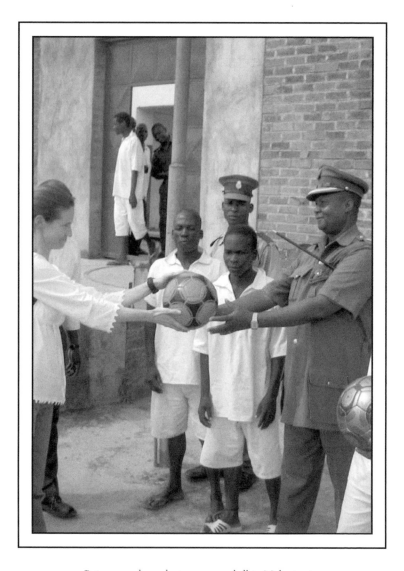

Prisoners and guards given a soccer ball in Malawi prison

39 Reform Prisons

PRISONS AROUND THE WORLD are ill-equipped to deal with HIV and AIDS. In Africa, facilities are so crowded that in order to change position while sleeping, one prisoner has to announce to the others to "roll over," and every man turns at the same time. In Latin America children go to jail with their parents. In the United States a high number of young African-American men are incarcerated for various periods of time, which may correlate with the disproportionate rate of HIV infections being experienced in the African American community.[3]

Most governments refuse to allow condom distribution in prisons, arguing it would encourage promiscuity. Yet sexual activity and abuse among prisoners remains rampant around the world. Overlooked and underfunded, correction facilities and programs fall at the low end of government and nongovernment priorities. Until prison reform turns an eye toward preventing the spread of HIV, the pandemic will continue.

IV.

_____

Yes, there must be more money
spent on this disease.
But there must also be a change in hearts and minds;
in cultures and attitudes.
Neither philanthropist nor scientist;
neither government nor church,
can solve this problem on their own—
AIDS must be an
all-hands-on-deck effort.

—Barack Obama

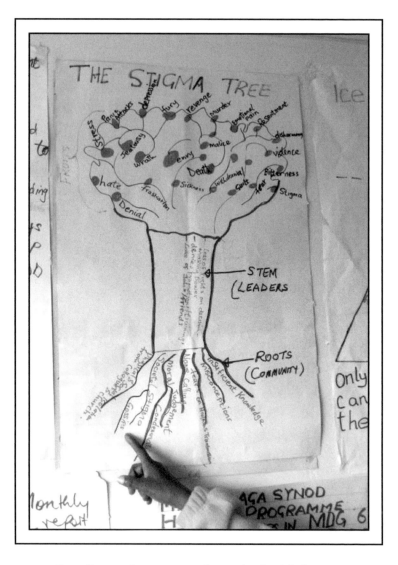

Poster illustrating how stigma contributes to denial and death in Kenya

40   Identify as HIV Positive

THE SINGER DIAMANDA GALÁS tattooed on her knuckles "We are all HIV+." To understand the dilemmas of and discrimination against persons with HIV and AIDS, we need to at least imagine, if not acknowledge, that we too are HIV positive. Instead of an us-and-them-perspective, let us attempt to enter into the world experienced daily by those living with HIV/AIDS. Far too many persons have lived—and died—with AIDS, having had to face alone the ugliness of discrimination and outright hatred. Some persons with AIDS have been rejected by their families. Some have been denied medical treatment and the companionship of their life partners. Young men in Panama have been dropped at hospitals by families who never return. Young mothers in Nepal have been tossed out of their homes and forced into commercial sex work. When we identify as HIV positive with these people, it signifies for us a major step away from condemnation to compassion, from exclusiveness to empathy.

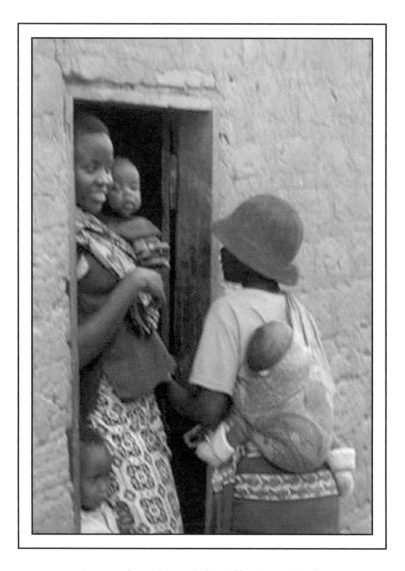

Young mothers visiting with their children in rural Zambia

41 Educate Girls and Young Women

A GIRL WITHOUT EDUCATION matures into a woman without a future. In many cultures, the probability is high that an uneducated girl will become infected with HIV barely beyond puberty. The lack of universal primary education means that females often end up staying at home, while their brothers get whatever education is available. As a consequence, illiteracy keeps a young girl from knowing even basic information about her body, health, sanitation, and diseases. The less education a girl has, the more babies she is likely to bear. Lack of family planning and birth control lead to HIV-positive mothers having more babies, even after one child tests positive. Educating girls now offers the possibility of healthier women and children in the future.

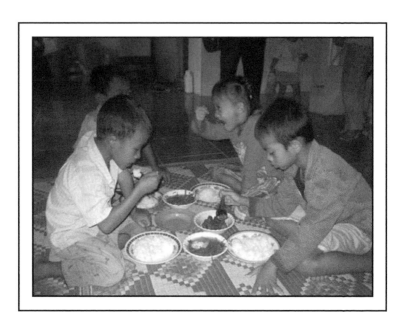

Cambodian AIDS orphans eating

42 Advocate an International School Lunch Program

IN BEAUTIFUL BUT IMPOVERISHED northern Malawi, a young educator shared his anguish that eighty-nine schools in the area, serving twenty-one thousand children, lacked a daily school lunch program. "Without at least one meal a day, the children are too listless to learn," he said. "Only the boys attend school; little girls stay home to work if there is food for them to eat." This young Malawian's words echo the counsel of two men he does not know of: former senators and presidential nominees George McGovern (Democrat of South Dakota) and Bob Dole (Republican of Kansas). Concerned about malnutrition and AIDS, these two senior statesmen long have advocated that the world would be healthier and more peaceful if children were fed daily at school. Children in school learn about disease and prevention. Advocating for U.S. expenditures through the McGovern-Dole International Food for Education and Child Nutrition Program advances the battle against HIV and AIDS.[4]

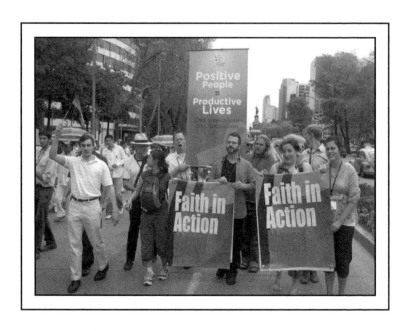

International March against Stigma, Discrimination, and Homophobia in Mexico

43 Lower Prices of Antiretroviral Medicines

HIV AND AIDS HAVE been called the "new apartheid" of the twenty-first century. In South Africa apartheid in the twentieth century meant lack of access to opportunities and institutions; today in southern Africa and elsewhere, the new apartheid means lack of access to life-sustaining but expensive antiretroviral medicines. Until recently, new AIDS patients in South Carolina had to wait for subsidized treatment until another patient died and freed up funds for them. In India a young man could afford medicine for only one of his infected parents and had to decide whom he would help live. Medical research is expensive, and corporations need fair compensation. But when faced with astronomical prices charged for these medicines by pharmaceutical companies, governments like Brazil and India have broken patent agreements to provide generics. Public pressure on these companies and negotiations by the Clinton Foundation and others have helped to lower the prices dramatically for certain countries. Even though prices have fallen to as low as $1 a day, millions of impoverished and infected persons cannot buy these miraculous tablets. The rock star Bono reminds us that "we have the drugs but we are not sharing them. I believe history and God will be our judge on this one."[5] Continued public protests to pharmaceutical companies and political action will help ensure access to these essential medicines.

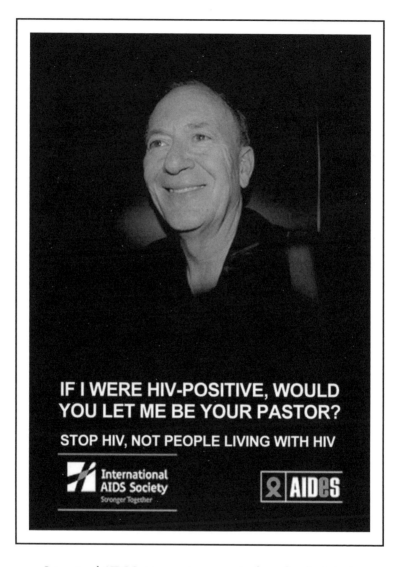

International AIDS Society campaign posters aimed at ending discrimination

44 Employ HIV-Positive Persons

WHEN PEOPLE FEAR losing their jobs if they test HIV positive, they often refuse to get tested and the virus continues to spread. Thanks to modern medicine, HIV and AIDS are manageable diseases; HIV-positive persons can live long and productive lives. Old prejudices, however, prevail. Ironically, even as former Secretary of State Condoleezza Rice led an effort against AIDS stigma and discrimination around the world, the U.S. Foreign Service automatically rejected applicants who were HIV positive. Only after one highly qualified applicant sued Condoleezza Rice and the State Department did the U.S. government lift its ban on allowing HIV-positive persons to join the Foreign Service. Creating an AIDS-free world means recognizing that employment discrimination is not only immoral but also should be illegal.

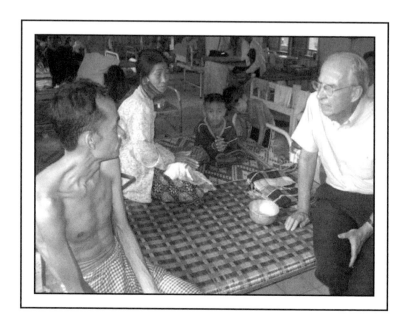

Visiting persons living with AIDS in Cambodia

45 Support the Global Fund

INDIVIDUAL CHARITIES PROVIDE invaluable works of mercy that governments and foundations often overlook or consider so small as not to be worth the paperwork. However, the massive AIDS crisis in the world also requires macroprograms of outreach. Initiated by former U.N. Secretary-General Kofi Annan, the Global Fund to Fight AIDS, Tuberculosis, and Malaria plays an indispensable role in mobilizing and monitoring government efforts around the world.[6] Because $10 billion a year is needed by this organization for prevention, care, and treatment, wealthy governments and corporations need to be encouraged to contribute regularly to this effort. Promises made by leaders of G-8 superpowers often are not kept, so citizen advocacy is essential. To paraphrase Winston Churchill, the treatment of the world's most impoverished citizens infected and affected by HIV and AIDS is one of the most unfailing tests of the civilization of any country.

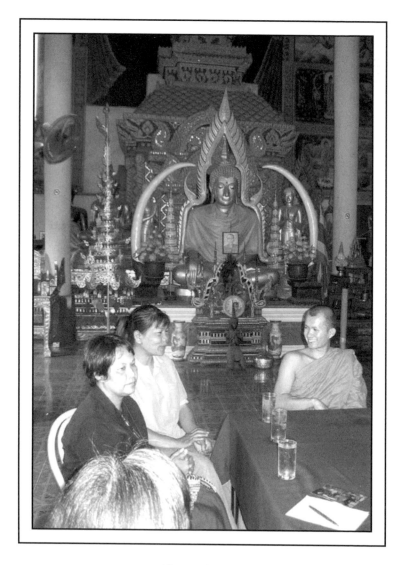

Buddhist temple in Thailand

46 Challenge Synagogue, Mosque, Church, Temple

WHEN MUSLIMS, CHRISTIANS, Jews, Buddhists, and Hindus came together for the first time in Bangkok for an International AIDS conference, Peter Piot, a physician and UNAIDS executive director, sketched a vision of his hopes. Piot declared,

> We hope for a day when: every church engages in open dialogue on issues of sexuality and gender difference; every synagogue mobilizes as advocates for global responses to fight HIV; every parish fully welcomes people who are HIV positive; every ashram understands and undertakes study and reflection on HIV; every pagoda is a place where young people learn the facts of HIV and AIDS; and every mosque is a safe place for seeking honest information on AIDS and referral to services.[7]

Faith communities alone cannot stop the global AIDS pandemic, but the pandemic cannot be stemmed without them.

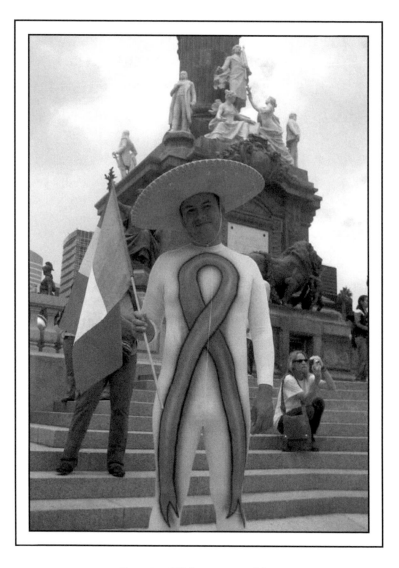

Promoting AIDS prevention in Mexico

47 Promote Circumcision

RESEARCH REVEALS THAT male circumcision reduces sexual transmission of HIV from women to men by about 60 percent. That fact has prompted many to line up for voluntary, safe, and informed surgeries. Others are less than eager to be on the cutting edge, however, since this is a painful prevention tool, fraught with cultural and religious controversy. Not a magic bullet, male circumcision does not provide total protection. The danger of increased risky male sexual behavior could offset the advantages, if persons avoid condoms or increase numbers of partners. Circumcision itself carries some risk. Many impoverished clinics and hospitals may have unsanitary methods, and anecdotal accounts of serious complications, including penile amputation, have been reported. Yet the world cannot ignore a 60 percent transmission reduction; this procedure could prove a powerful tool to curb HIV. Scientists speculate that promoting circumcision in sub-Saharan Africa could avert up to 5.7 million new HIV infections and more than three million deaths over the next twenty years.

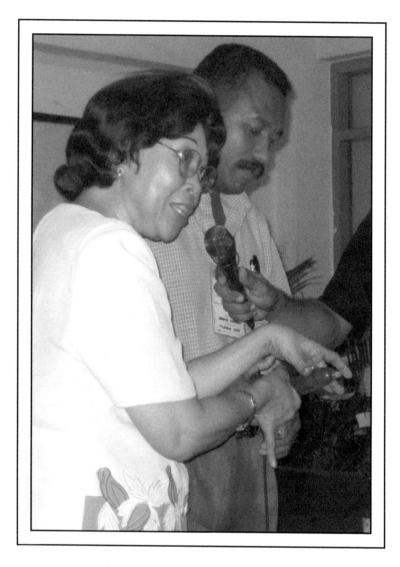

Indonesian physician demonstrates AIDS prevention

48 Lubricate

IN JAKARTA, INDONESIA, a questioner in the audience asked, "Why is dry sex dangerous?" An Indonesian female physician quickly responded, warning that dry sex as practiced in various countries can be exceedingly unsafe. Zimbabwean women dry out their vaginas with *mutendo wegudo*—soil contaminated with baboon urine—while others use detergents, salt, cotton or shredded newspaper. Sub-Saharan African men often demand that women have dry and tight vaginas, which makes sex painful for the woman. Dry sex destroys natural antiseptic moisture protection, which increases vaginal tearing, rips condoms, and escalates the chances for sexually transmitted diseases including HIV. These practices have helped inflame the pandemic in the region. Lubrication becomes more and more important as people age. Lubricate for safer sex whether in Nairobi, Nanjing, or Nashville.

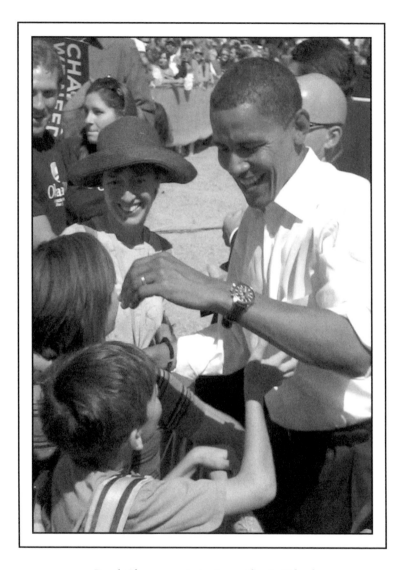

Barack Obama campaigning for president in Colorado

49 Vote for Candidates Who Care

AIDS CANNOT BE CONQUERED without political leadership. The pandemic took off throughout the world because politicians in country after country lived in denial and failed to act quickly. Still many give only lip service to upgrading health services and promoting prevention. Individuals can make a difference both by voting for candidates who care and by holding them accountable when in office. Too often critical domestic AIDS programs like the Ryan White CARE Act do not receive sufficient monies. In 2003 President George W. Bush proposed a $15 billion dollar, five-year program to combat AIDS in Africa and the Caribbean. Thanks to bipartisan support in 2008, PEPFAR (President's Emergency Plan for AIDS Relief) received reauthorization for five years at $50 billion. Financial figures of that magnitude are hard to grasp. But among the millions of people being helped is a young Kenyan mother. Rose's husband had died; she was sick and awaiting the angel of death. She expected her children would soon be orphaned with no one to care for them. But American antiretroviral medical help arrived, and she now is a productive parent and citizen, serving as an assistant manager of a farm. How much better it is to keep parents alive than to build more orphanages. Let our votes count on the side of life!

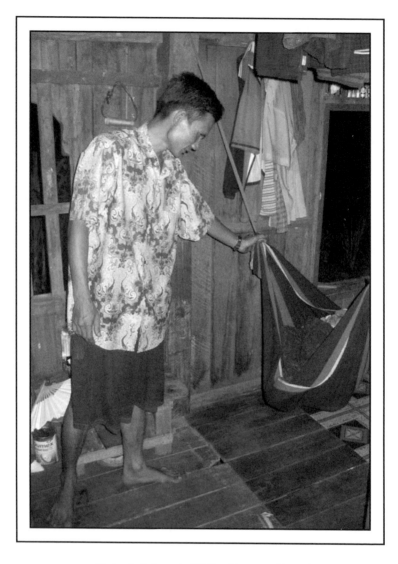

Caring for baby with AIDS in Myanmar (Burma)

50 Reduce the Craving for Dangerous Drugs

THE USE AND ABUSE of heroin and other dangerous drugs proves to be a major factor in the spread of HIV in the world. In the remote Xinjiang region of China on the edge of the Gobi Desert, AIDS is rampant among poor Muslims of Turkic descent known as the Uyghurs because of using shared dirty needles while injecting heroin. About 30 percent are infected with HIV—with the highest rates of reported prevalence among injecting drug users anywhere in the world. In the United States the percentage of HIV infection for injecting drug users is about 5 percent for whites, 8 percent among Hispanics, and 12 percent in the African-American community. Exceptionally high rates of infection also are evident near the Golden Triangle, an opium-growing area that includes Myanmar (Burma), Laos, and Thailand, with an overflow of the pandemic into Northeast India. Efforts are underway to curtail the craving for heroin through the use of Suboxone, a drug that appears safer to prescribe than methadone, the standard heroin detoxification drug. What helps to create an AIDS-free world are government programs that offer clean needle exchanges, subsidize detoxification drugs, and provide rehabilitation programs. Call, e-mail, or write your elected representatives about this need. Politicians often refuse to support these programs, despite their life-giving benefits, unless they receive support and encouragement from their voting constituents.

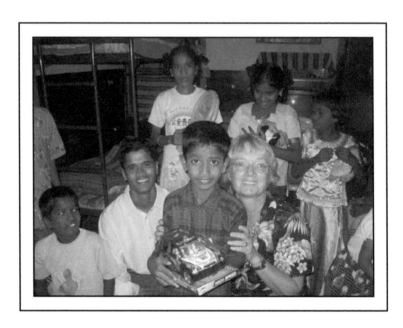

Sharing toys at an AIDS orphanage in India

51 Do One Thing

SOMEONE HAS NOTED there are 145,394,726 great needs in this world. If you try to deal with all of them, you will collapse. No one person can save the world, as the challenge is too big and overwhelming. Choose, however, at least one great need to champion and work on it. People as diverse as Bono, Mother Teresa, and the Dalai Lama have stressed the significance of one person's action. Most change does not happen in one year, but it is astounding how much change can occur in ten years. By implementing the fifty-two ways highlighted in this book we can make a difference not only in our personal arenas but throughout the entire world. Embrace with passionate commitment at least one task in helping create an AIDS-free world—like helping orphans in Malawi, getting medicine to mothers at childbirth in India, or educating girls in Honduras. Encourage others to pick up one of the other 145,394,725 needs!

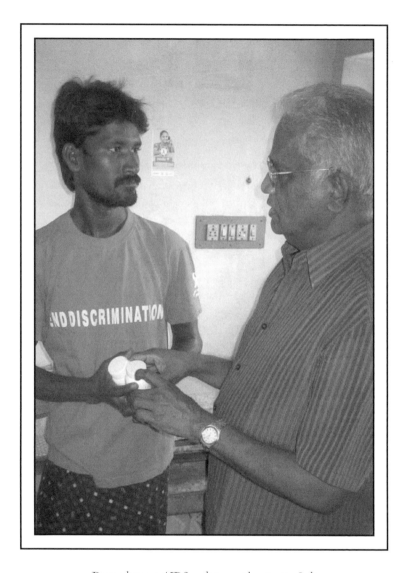

Doctor discusses AIDS medicines with patient in India

52 Let an AIDS-Free World Begin with Me

WITHOUT A PERSONAL COMMITMENT to end AIDS, the other fifty-one ways outlined in this book are unlikely to stop the pandemic. All the public health slogans in the world ultimately fail unless matched by actions reflecting personal responsibility. Whether this means stating bluntly to "stop screwing around"[8], as Larry Kramer did, or a renewed vow to avoid behavior clearly marked by danger signs, we take steps to couple personal freedom with individual accountability. Some persons—like men incarcerated in violent prisons and women in oppressive relationships or cultures—may lack choice, but where freedom exists, individuals are called to exercise conviction, control, courage, and commitment. As Gandhi once said, "We need to be the change we wish to see in the world."[9] An AIDS-free world will not just happen.

Resources for Action and Information

Web Sites

www.unaids.org
www.churchandglobalaids.org
www.pedaids.org
www.umglobalaidsfund.org
www.avert.org
www.hivforum.org
www.gmhc.org
www.projectinform.org
www.healthgap.org
www.globalstrategies.org
www.stopglobalaids.org
www.stophungernow.org
www.careusa.org
www.bread.org
www.secondharvest.org
www.alliancetoendhunger.org

Books

Ammicht-Quinn, Regina and Hille Hacker, eds. *Concilium: AIDS* 2007, no. 3.

Bono, *On the Move.* Nashville, TN: Thomas Nelson, 2007.

Bourke, Dale Hanson. *The Skeptic's Guide to the Global AIDS Crisis: Tough Questions Direct Answers,* Rev. ed. Tyrone, GA: Authentic Publishing, 2006.

D'Adesky, Anne-Christine. *Moving Mountains: The Race to Treat Global AIDS.* New York: Verso Books, 2006.

Epstein, Helen. *The Invisible Cure: Why We Are Losing the Fight against AIDS in Africa.* New York: Picador, 2008.

Farmer, Paul, Margaret Connors, and Janie Simmons, eds. *Women, Poverty and AIDS: Sex, Drugs and Structural Violence.* Monroe, ME: Common Courage Press, 2005.

Gill, Peter. *The Politics of AIDS: How They Turned a Disease into a Disaster.* New Delhi: Viva Books Private Limited, 2007.

Green, Edward C. *Rethinking AIDS Prevention: Learning from Successes in Developing Countries.* Portsmouth, NH: Greenwood Publishing, 2003.

Kidder, Tracy. *Mountains Beyond Mountains: The Quest of Dr. Paul Farmer, a Man Who Would Cure the World.* New York: Random House, 2009.

McGovern, George S., Bob Dole, and Donald E. Messer, *Ending Hunger Now: A Challenge to Persons of Faith.* Minneapolis, MN: Augsburg Fortress, Publishers, 2005.

Messer, Donald E. *Breaking the Conspiracy of Silence: Christian Churches and the Global AIDS Crisis.* Minneapolis, MN: Augsburg Fortress, Publishers, 2004.

Mutti, Fritz and Etta Mae. *Dancing in a Wheelchair: One Family Faces HIV/AIDS.* Nashville, TN: Abingdon Press, 2004.

Steinberg, Jonny. *Three Letter Plague.* London: Random House, 2009.

Tucker, Neely. *Love in the Driest Season: A Family Memoir.* New York: Three Rivers Press/Crown Publishing, 2005.

Notes

1. Muhammad Yunus, *Creating a World without Poverty: Social Business and the Future of Capitalism*, with Karl Weber. (New York: PublicAffairs, 2007), 223.

2. Julio Montaner, M.D., quoted in Rod Mickleburgh, "More HIV Treatment Could Cut Subsequent Cases 60 Per Cent," *Globe and Mail* (July 3, 2008).

3. See http://www.caps.ucsf.edu/pubs/FS/inmaterev.php for a fact sheet on the role of prisons in HIV prevention.

4. For information about the McGovern-Dole International Food for Education and Child Nutrition Program, see http://www.friendsofwfp.org/site/pp.asp?c=7oIJLSOsGpF&b=2048389

5. BBC World News Service, *Bono: World AIDS Day 2002, Part 2*, BBCi, December 2002, http://www.bbc.co.uk/.

6. Find out how to contribute to the Global Fund to Fight AIDS, Tuberculosis and Malaria at http:/www.theglobalfund.org/EN/

7. Peter Piot, UNAIDS Executive Director, speech at the Ecumenical Gathering "Access for All: The Faith Community Responding," Bangkok, July 10, 2004. See http://data.unaids.org/pub/Speech/2004/sp_piot_interfaith_10jul04_en.pdf

8. See Larry Kramer's blunt speech of November 7, 2004, at http://towleroad.typepad.com/towleroad/2004/11/larry_kramer_sp.html

9. Mahatma Gandhi, quoted in Michel W. Potts, "Arun Gandhi Shares the Mahatma's Message," in *India-West* (San Leandro, CA) 27, no. 13 (1 February 2002): A34; Arun Gandhi is indirectly quoting his grandfather. See also "Be the Change You Wish to See: An Interview with Arun Gandhi," in Carmella O'Hahn, *Reclaiming Children and Youth* (Bloomington) 10, no. 1 (Spring 2001): 6.

HIV and AIDS Are Preventable Diseases

LET'S BE CLEAR; unlike many other diseases, HIV and AIDS are preventable diseases. No one should accept the inevitability of an AIDS pandemic because steps can be taken to protect oneself and others from this virus. An AIDS-free world requires avoiding risky personal behavior and working to create societies where persons are liberated from inequality, illiteracy, violence, and poverty.

Completely "safe sex" proves to be an impossibility, but persons can practice "safer sex," minimizing the possibilities of becoming infected or of infecting others. The probabilities of infection from unprotected anal or vaginal sex are considerably higher than from unprotected oral sex, but a small degree of possibility exists.

Be cautious. Remember most people infected with HIV do not look sick, and a large percentage of persons who are HIV positive have never been tested and do not know they are infected.

You Could Get Infected by:

*   Engaging in unprotected vaginal, anal, or oral sex with a person who already has the virus. Protection requires the consistent and correct use of condoms, remembering that condoms can be defective or break in use.

- Sharing needles when shooting drugs with a person already infected.
- Having open skin wounds exposed to infected semen, blood, or urine.
- Getting blood or blood products that have been contaminated by the virus.
- Passing the virus from an infected mother to her baby during pregnancy, delivery, or during breast-feeding.
- Experiencing deep mouth-to-mouth wet kissing with an infected person, if you have mouth sores or bleeding gums.
- Reusing condoms, sharing dildos or other sex toys.
- Tattooing and body piercing with unsterilized equipment used previously on an infected person.

You Cannot Get Infected by:

- Contact through handshaking; hugging; touching; sneezing; eating utensils; musical instruments; or sharing swimming pools, showers, washing facilities, or toilet seats.
- Dry kissing, massage, or insect bites.
- Solo or mutual masturbation.
- Abstinence from sex.
- Using sterile needles.
- Enjoying sex with an uninfected partner.

The Terminology of HIV and AIDS

CERTAIN WORDS AND ACRONYMS are commonly used when discussing the global HIV and AIDS crisis. Check Web sites for additional information.

HIV stands for human immunodeficiency virus. Immunodeficiency refers to the decline of the body's immune system to resist infection and disease.

AIDS represents acquired immunodeficiency syndrome, meaning it is something you get, not a genetic disease that weakens your immune system. Technically AIDS is not a single disease since AIDS patients usually have many diseases, each with its own signs and symptoms. From a scientific perspective, people do not die from AIDS but from other opportunistic infections, cancers, and organ failures triggered by an inadequate immune system.

ARV or antiretroviral drugs stop or reduce HIV from reproducing inside the body, strengthening the immune system's ability to fight infections.

CSW (commercial sex workers), an internationally used term for male or female workers and a less derogatory word than *prostitutes*. The term emphasizes the fact that persons are employed in this way for financial reasons, many engaged in "survival sex" to feed their families.

MSM refers to men who have sex with men, rather than speaking of gay or bisexual males.

Microbicides are gels, creams, or foams used to destroy bacteria or viruses. Research is underway to discover vaginal and anal microbicides that would reduce HIV infection.

Pandemic emphasizes the global nature of a widely spread disease versus epidemic, which tends to be more regional or isolated.

Harm reduction reflects a public health philosophy and pragmatic strategy that seeks to minimize and reduce negative consequences from drug usage, alcohol, and sexual behaviors, without demanding total abstinence as a starting point. Abstinence-based strategies, however, are an integral component of comprehensive harm reduction.

Evidence-based prevention emphasizes using scientifically verified approaches to HIV and AIDS prevention, not simply accenting religious values or ideological statements. Controversy particularly revolves around abstinence-only programs versus comprehensive sexuality education.

About the Author

DONALD E. MESSER is executive director of the Center for the Church and Global AIDS, as well as President Emeritus and Henry White Warren Professor Emeritus of Practical Theology at the Iliff School of Theology, Denver, Colorado.

The author of fifteen books, Messer has received outstanding alumni awards from Boston University and Dakota Wesleyan University and in 2008 was named to the South Dakota Hall of Fame.